BREAKING PANCREATIC SILENCE

CURING THE CORE

JACOB WILLIAMS

Copyright

Table of Contents

Chapter 1: Introduction and Epidemiology

Introduction

Pancreatic cancer is one of the most formidable malignancies in oncology, characterized by late diagnosis, rapid progression, and limited treatment options. Although it ranks lower in incidence compared to other major cancers, such as breast, lung, or colorectal cancer,ncreatic cancer is consistently among the top causes of cancer-related mortality worldwide. Its lethality is often attributed to its asymptomatic nature in the early stages, aggressive tumor biology, and resistance to conventional therapies.

In the past two decades, there has been a growing focus on pancreatic cancer owing to its rising incidence and disproportionately high mortality rate. Numerous international health organizations and research institutions have prioritized it as a critical area of unmet medical need. Understanding its epidemiology, risk factors, and demographic distribution is vital for clinicians, researchers, and public health professionals engaged in early detection, prevention, and management strategies.

This chapter explores the burden of pancreatic cancer globally, the known risk factors, and trends in its epidemiology, with an emphasis on how these data inform clinical and research efforts aimed at improving outcomes.

Global Incidence and Mortality

Pancreatic cancer is the **seventh leading cause of cancer-related death globally**, accounting for more than 495,000 new cases and over 466,000 deaths annually (Global Cancer Observatory, 2020). These figures translate into a nearly 94% mortality-to-incidence ratio, underscoring the aggressive nature of this malignancy.

Regional Variation

The incidence of pancreatic cancer shows substantial geographical variation. High-income countries such as the United States, Canada, Japan, and several European nations exhibit the highest incidence rates. In contrast, the lowest rates are observed in parts of Africa and South Asia. This disparity is often linked to differences in lifestyle risk factors, diagnostic infrastructure, aging populations, and healthcare access.

Gender and Age Disparity

Pancreatic cancer affects both men and women, although incidence is slightly higher in males. It is predominantly a disease of older adults, with most diagnoses occurring in individuals aged 60 years and older. The median age at diagnosis in the United States is approximately 71 years.

Trends Over Time

Despite advances in medical technology, **5-year survival rates for pancreatic cancer remain dismally low—typically below 10%** in most countries. While the incidence of some cancers like colorectal or cervical has decreased due to successful screening and prevention efforts, pancreatic cancer has shown a **gradual but steady increase** in incidence over the last few decades.

Survival Trends

Recent years have seen a marginal improvement in short-term survival, mainly due to better surgical techniques, improved perioperative care, and modest gains in chemotherapy regimens. However, these improvements have not significantly shifted long-term survival.

Projected Burden

Epidemiological models project that pancreatic cancer will become the **second leading cause of cancer-related death** in the United States by 2030 if current trends continue. Similar projections have been made in Europ and East Asia, emphasizing the urgency of focused intervention strategies.

Risk Factors

A better understanding of pancreatic cancer risk factors is crucial for developing prevention and early detection strategies. These risk factors are broadly categorized into **modifiable** and **non-modifiable** types.

Modifiable Risk Factors

- **Tobacco Use**: Cigarette smoking is the most well-established environmental risk factor, doubling the risk of pancreatic cancer. Approximately 20–25% of pancreatic cancer cases are attributable to smoking.
- **Obesity and Diet**: A high body mass index (BMI) and a diet rich in red and processed meats are associated with

an increased risk, likely due to chronic inflammation and insulin resistance.

- **Alcohol Consumption**: Chronic heavy alcohol use can lead to pancreatitis, a known risk factor for pancreatic cancer.

- **Occupational Exposures**: Prolonged exposure to certain industrial chemicals such as petroleum derivatives and pesticides has been linked to a modest increase in risk.

Non-modifiable Risk Factors

- **Age**: The incidence increases significantly after the age of 50, peaking in the seventh and eighth decades of life.

- **Genetics and Family History**: Individuals with a first-degree relative who has had pancreatic cancer have a two to threefold increased risk. Approximately 10% of cases have a hereditary component.

- **Genetic Syndromes**: Several hereditary syndromes are associated with a higher risk, including:

  - Hereditary Pancreatitis (PRSS1 mutations)
  - Peutz-Jeghers Syndrome (STK11 mutation)
  - Lynch Syndrome (MMR gene mutations)

- ○ BRCA1 and BRCA2 mutations, especially in Ashkenazi Jewish populations
- **Chronic Pancreatitis**: Long-standing inflammation of the pancreas significantly increases cancer risk, particularly in cases linked to hereditary causes or autoimmune pancreatitis.

- **Diabetes Mellitus**: Long-standing diabetes, particularly type 2, is associated with increased risk, although the relationship may be bidirectional.

Screening and Early Detection

Currently, there is **no validated population-wide screening test** for pancreatic cancer, mainly due to the lack of sensitive and specific biomarkers and the deep anatomical location of the pancreas. However, research is underway to develop risk-based screening models, particularly for individuals with a strong family history or genetic predisposition.

- **High-Risk Groups**: Screening may be considered
  in individuals with two or more first-degree relatives affected or in those carrying known pathogenic mutations. Modalities such as endoscopic ultrasound (EUS) and magnetic resonance cholangiopancreatography (MRCP) are being explored.

- **Biomarkers**: CA 19-9 is the most commonly used biomarker but has low sensitivity in early disease and can be elevated in benign conditions. Novel biomarkers like circulating tumor DNA (ctDNA) and exosomal proteins are under investigation.

Socioeconomic and Racial Disparities

Health disparities play a significant role in the outcomes of pancreatic cancer:

- **Racial Disparities**: In the United States, African Americans have a higher incidence and worse survival compared to Caucasians, possibly due to differences in access to care, socioeconomic factors, and biological factors.

- **Socioeconomic Status**: Lower socioeconomic
  status is correlated with delayed diagnosis, limited access to specialized care, and poorer outcomes. Rural populations are particularly vulnerable due to the scarcity of high-volume surgical centers.

- **Global Inequities**: In low- and middle-income countries (LMICs), limited diagnostic infrastructure and lack of trained specialists delay diagnosis and treatment, leading to disproportionately high mortality rates.

The Public Health Challenge

Pancreatic cancer represents a **complex public health challenge** due to its silent progression, lack of early detection tools, and poor response to treatment. Public health efforts must focus on:

- **Raising Awareness**: Educating healthcare providers and the public about early symptoms and risk factors.
- **Improving Access**: Enhancing access to diagnostic imaging, biopsy procedures, and specialized cancer centers.
- **Funding Research**: Increasing investment in basic science and translational research to discover effective biomarkers, therapeutic targets, and screening protocols.
- **Registry Data**: Establishing and maintaining comprehensive cancer registries, especially in underserved

regions, to better understand epidemiologic patterns.

Chapter 2: Anatomy and Pathophysiology of the Pancreas

Introduction

A comprehensive understanding of the pancreas's anatomical structure and physiological function is essential in grasping the pathogenesis, diagnosis, and management of pancreatic cancer. The pancreas plays a vital role in both the digestive and endocrine systems, and its complex location and ductal network make surgical and medical management particularly challenging.

In this chapter, we will explore the macro- and microscopic anatomy of the pancreas, its physiological functions, and the pathological mechanisms that drive pancreatic tumorigenesis, with a focus on the molecular alterations characteristic of pancreatic ductal adenocarcinoma (PDAC)—the most common form of pancreatic cancer.

Gross Anatomy of the Pancreas

The pancreas is a **retroperitoneal organ** located in the upper abdomen. It lies transversely across the posterior abdominal wall and is closely related to several vital structures, including the duodenum, stomach, spleen, and major blood vessels such as the superior mesenteric artery

(SMA), superior mesenteric vein (SMV), portal vein, and celiac trunk.

Anatomical Divisions

The pancreas is divided into five main parts:

- **Head**: Nestled within the curvature of the duodenum; this is the most common site of pancreatic tumors.
- **Uncinate Process**: A small hook-like extension of the head that wraps around the SMA and SMV.
- **Neck**: Lies anterior to the SMV and portal vein confluence.

- **Body**: Extends to the left, crossing the aorta and lying posterior to the stomach.
- **Tail**: Terminates near the splenic hilum and is closely associated with the spleen.

Ductal System

The pancreatic ductal system includes:

- **Main Pancreatic Duct (Wirsung)**: Joins the common bile duct to form the hepatopancreatic ampulla (of Vater), which drains into the duodenum.
- **Accessory Duct (Santorini)**: Drains part of the head and opens separately into the duodenum.

Tumors originating near the ampulla may present early with jaundice due to biliary obstruction, while those in the tail often remain asymptomatic until advanced.

Microscopic Anatomy and Cellular Composition

The pancreas contains two major components:

- **Exocrine pancreas**: Comprising about 85% of the pancreatic tissue, it includes acinar cells that produce digestive enzymes and a ductal system for enzyme transport.

- **Endocrine pancreas**: Comprising the islets of Langerhans, it regulates glucose metabolism through hormone secretion.

Acinar Cells

These cells produce digestive enzymes such as amylase, lipase, and proteases. Chronic inflammation in acinar tissue, such as from pancreatitis, may predispose to malignant transformation.

Ductal Cells

The ductal epithelium lines the pancreatic ducts and is the origin of most pancreatic cancers, particularly PDAC.

Islets of Langerhans

These endocrine clusters secrete insulin, glucagon, somatostatin, and pancreatic polypeptide. Neuroendocrine tumors (PNETs) arise from these cells but differ significantly from ductal adenocarcinomas in presentation and prognosis.

Physiology of the Pancreas

The pancreas plays dual roles:

- **Exocrine Function**: Digestive enzymes are secreted into the duodenum to assist in digestion.
- **Endocrine Function**: Hormones regulate blood glucose and metabolism.

Enzymatic Function

Acinar cells are stimulated by cholecystokinin (CCK) and vagal activity to release enzymes. Pancreatic secretions are alkaline due to bicarbonate production by ductal cells, helping neutralize gastric acid in the duodenum.

Hormonal Regulation

Key hormones secreted include:

- **Insulin** (beta cells): Lowers blood glucose.

- **Glucagon** (alpha cells): Raises blood glucose.
- **Somatostatin** (delta cells): Inhibits insulin and glucagon.
- **Pancreatic Polypeptide**: Regulates pancreatic secretions.

Pathophysiology of Pancreatic Cancer

The majority of pancreatic malignancies (approximately 90%) are **pancreatic ductal adenocarcinomas (PDAC)**, originating from the epithelial lining of the ducts.

Carcinogenesis

Pancreatic cancer develops through a stepwise accumulation of genetic mutations in precursor lesions:

- **PanIN (Pancreatic Intraepithelial Neoplasia)**:
    Microscopic lesions in ductal epithelium.

- **IPMN (Intraductal Papillary Mucinous Neoplasm)**: Grossly visible mucin-producing lesions.
- **MCN (Mucinous Cystic Neoplasm)**: Occur
    predominantly in women and typically in the tail.

Progression involves histological changes from low-grade dysplasia to high-grade dysplasia and ultimately to invasive carcinoma.

Molecular and Genetic Alterations

Key Genetic Mutations

- **KRAS**: Mutated in >90% of PDAC cases; promotes uncontrolled cell proliferation.
- **TP53**: Tumor suppressor gene mutation leads to evasion of apoptosis.

- **CDKN2A/p16**: Regulates cell cycle; loss leads to unchecked progression from G1 to S phase.
- **SMAD4**: Loss of this gene disrupts TGF-β signaling and is associated with poor prognosis.

Epigenetic Changes

Alterations in DNA methylation, histone modification, and non-coding RNA expression also play a role in tumorigenesis.

Tumor Microenvironment

The pancreatic tumor microenvironment is rich in:

- **Desmoplastic Stroma**: Dense fibrotic tissue that impairs drug delivery.
- **Immune Cells**: Tumors evade immune surveillance via regulatory T-cells and myeloid-derived suppressor cells (MDSCs).
- **Hypoxia**: Low oxygen levels within the tumor lead to aggressive phenotypes and therapy resistance.

Tumor Spread and Metastasis

PDAC is characterized by early and aggressive local invasion and distant metastasis.

Local Invasion

- The proximity to critical vascular structures (e.g., portal vein, SMA) facilitates direct extension, often making the tumor unresectable at diagnosis.

Perineural Invasion

. A hallmark of pancreatic cancer, contributing to severe abdominal and back pain and increased local recurrence after surgery.

Hematogenous Spread

Common metastatic sites include:

- **Liver** (most frequent)
- **Lungs** • **Peritoneum**
- **Bones** (less common)

Clinical Implications of Anatomy and Pathophysiology

Diagnostic Challenges

The deep retroperitoneal location and nonspecific early symptoms hinder early detection. Anatomical knowledge is essential when interpreting imaging studies and planning biopsies or surgery.

Surgical Considerations

Resection feasibility depends heavily on tumor location and vascular involvement:

- Tumors in the **head** are addressed with pancreaticoduodenectomy (Whipple procedure).
- Tumors in the **tail** may require distal pancreatectomy with splenectomy.

- Involvement of the **SMA or celiac axis** usually indicates unresectability.

Treatment Resistance

The desmoplastic stroma not only impedes drug delivery but also fosters a protective niche for tumor cells, reducing the effectiveness of chemotherapy and immunotherapy.

Emerging Areas in Pathophysiology

Organoid Models

Patient-derived organoids are being developed to study tumor behavior and test drugs ex vivo.

Circulating Tumor Cells (CTCs) and DNA (ctDNA)

These biomarkers may aid in early detection and monitoring treatment response.

Immunopathology

The immune-evasive nature of PDAC is an area of intense research, with focus on overcoming T-cell exclusion and stromal suppression to enhance immunotherapy efficacy.

Chapter 3

Clinical Presentation and Diagnosis

Pancreatic cancer remains one of the most lethal malignancies globally due to its late presentation and limited options for curative treatment. Unlike cancers of the breast or colon, which benefit from established screening protocols, pancreatic cancer often progresses silently until symptoms indicate advanced disease. A thorough understanding of its clinical manifestations and the diagnostic process is crucial for clinicians to detect it early, identify high-risk individuals, and initiate timely management.

This chapter provides a comprehensive exploration of the signs and symptoms associated with pancreatic cancer, the diagnostic approaches—including imaging, laboratory tests, tissue sampling—and staging frameworks that guide treatment decisions.

Clinical Manifestations of Pancreatic Cancer

The clinical presentation of pancreatic cancer is often subtle, non-specific, and easily misattributed to more benign gastrointestinal conditions. These symptoms vary depending on the **anatomical location** of the tumor—whether it arises in the **head**, **body**, or **tail** of the pancreas.

Tumors of the Head of the Pancreas

Tumors in the head region frequently result in **biliary obstruction** due to their proximity to the common bile duct. Patients often present with **painless jaundice**, which includes symptoms such as yellowing of the skin and eyes, dark urine, pale stools, and generalized pruritus. The classic **Courvoisier's sign**, which refers to a palpable, non-tender gallbladder in the setting of obstructive jaundice, is occasionally appreciated in physical exams.

Other manifestations may include vague **epigastric pain**, especially postprandial or radiating to the back, along with **nausea**, **early satiety**, and **weight loss**.

Tumors of the Body and Tail

Lesions in the body or tail of the pancreas tend to remain asymptomatic until they invade adjacent structures or metastasize.

Symptoms often include **dull abdominal pain**, **back pain**, or **significant weight loss**. At this stage, the disease is frequently inoperable. **New-onset diabetes mellitus**, particularly in individuals over the age of 50 with no prior metabolic disorder, may be an early indicator of a developing neoplasm in these locations.

Systemic and Paraneoplastic Features

In addition to local symptoms, pancreatic cancer may manifest systemically:

- **Anorexia and Cachexia**:
  Unexplained and severe weight loss is

common and often related to both metabolic effects of the tumor and systemic inflammation.

- **Venous Thromboembolism**: Pancreatic cancer is highly thrombotic. Patients may present with **deep vein thrombosis (DVT)** or the more rare **Trousseau's syndrome**— a migratory thrombophlebitis.
- **Fatigue and Malaise**: Non-specific but common, these symptoms reflect systemic involvement.
- **Depression**: Some studies suggest that mood changes may precede diagnosis, likely mediated by cytokines or neuroendocrine effects.

Approach to Clinical Diagnosis

Timely diagnosis hinges on a structured clinical evaluation, which includes a thorough history, targeted physical examination, and prompt initiation of appropriate investigations.

Physical Examination

Physical findings may be subtle or absent in the early stages. In advanced disease, one might observe:

- **Icterus** (jaundice), especially in tumors of the pancreatic head.
- **Palpable mass** in the epigastrium.
- **Hepatomegaly** or **ascites**, indicative of liver metastasis or peritoneal spread.

- **Virchow's node** (enlarged left supraclavicular lymph node) in cases of advanced malignancy.

Laboratory Investigations

Tumor Markers

- **CA 19-9**: The most widely used marker, elevated in approximately 70-80% of patients. While not useful for screening, it is valuable for monitoring response to therapy. However, false positives may occur in benign conditions such as cholangitis, and false negatives in Lewis antigen-negative individuals (~5% of the population).

- **CEA (Carcinoembryonic Antigen)**: Less specific but may complement CA 19-9 in diagnosis.

Liver Function Tests

Elevated **bilirubin, alkaline phosphatase**, and **transaminases** may signal biliary obstruction.

Metabolic Panels

Check for **hyperglycemia** or new-onset **diabetes mellitus**.

Radiological and Endoscopic Imaging

Imaging plays a pivotal role in detecting the primary tumor, assessing resectability, and staging metastases.

Abdominal Ultrasound

Often the first imaging modality used in jaundiced patients. It can detect biliary tree dilation and sometimes identify mass lesions, though its utility is limited by body habitus and operator dependency.

Contrast-Enhanced CT (Pancreatic Protocol)

The **gold standard** for initial imaging, it provides high-resolution details of the pancreas, surrounding vessels, lymph nodes, and liver metastasis. It is also crucial in evaluating vascular invasion which determines surgical resectability.

MRI and MRCP

MRI offers superior soft tissue contrast and is especially helpful in evaluating cystic lesions. MRCP provides non-invasive visualization of the pancreatic and bile ducts.

Endoscopic Ultrasound (EUS)

EUS is superior for identifying small tumors and allows for **fine needle aspiration (FNA)** to obtain tissue for histological diagnosis. It is highly sensitive and specific and is preferred when other imaging modalities are inconclusive.

PET-CT

Useful in detecting occult metastatic disease not apparent on CT or MRI, although not routinely performed.

Histological Confirmation

Tissue diagnosis is essential before initiating systemic therapy, especially in advanced or borderline resectable disease.

Fine Needle Aspiration (FNA)

Performed via EUS or CT guidance, FNA allows cytologic evaluation to confirm malignancy.

Core Biopsy

Obtains a larger tissue sample for molecular and immunohistochemical analysis, necessary for precision oncology.

In resectable tumors, some centers proceed directly to surgery without a biopsy, particularly when radiographic findings are definitive.

Staging of Pancreatic Cancer

Staging is essential to guide treatment and involves the **TNM classification**:

- **T (Tumor)**: Size and extent of invasion into adjacent structures.
- **N (Nodes)**: Involvement of regional lymph nodes.
- **M (Metastases)**: Distant organ involvement, especially the liver, lungs, and peritoneum.

Based on imaging and staging, tumors are classified as:

- **Resectable**: No vascular involvement or distant metastasis.
- **Borderline Resectable**: Limited encasement of mesenteric vessels.
- **Locally Advanced**: Involves major vessels, not amenable to resection.
- **Metastatic**: Spread beyond the pancreas.

Genetic and Molecular Diagnostics

In recent years, genomic testing has assumed a central role in managing pancreatic cancer.

- **Germline Testing** is recommended for all patients, particularly for BRCA1/2 mutations, which may respond to PARP inhibitors.
- **Somatic Tumor Profiling** can uncover actionable mutations (e.g., KRAS wild-type or mismatch repair deficiencies) that inform targeted therapies.

- **Microsatellite Instability (MSI)** and **dMMR** testing guide the use of immunotherapies like checkpoint inhibitors in rare but actionable subtypes.

Diagnostic Challenges

Diagnosing pancreatic cancer is fraught with difficulties:

- **Non-specific Symptoms**: Often mimic benign gastrointestinal conditions.

- **Lack of Early Detection Tools**: No effective screening tests for the general population.
- **Late Presentation**: By the time symptoms develop, many tumors are inoperable.
- **Overlap with Pancreatitis**: Distinguishing cancer from chronic pancreatitis can be difficult, even with advanced imaging.

Certainly! Below is **Chapter 4: Surgical Management of Pancreatic Cancer** from your book *"Management of Pancreatic Cancer"*. This chapter is structured in a **book format** with standard subheadings. Headings are to be styled in **font size 20**, and the main body text in **font size 14**, with a total word count exceeding 1400 words to meet your requirement.

Chapter 4

Surgical Management of Pancreatic Cancer

Surgical intervention remains the only potentially curative treatment for pancreatic cancer. Despite advances in chemotherapy, immunotherapy, and precision medicine, surgery remains the cornerstone of long-term survival, particularly for patients diagnosed at a stage where complete resection is possible. However, only about 15–20% of patients present with resectable disease at the time of diagnosis. The goal of surgical treatment is complete removal of the tumor (R0 resection) while minimizing perioperative morbidity and mortality.

This chapter provides a comprehensive analysis of surgical indications, types of pancreatic resections, preoperative evaluation, intraoperative considerations, postoperative care, and outcomes associated with pancreatic cancer surgery.

Indications for Surgical Resection

Surgical resection is considered in patients with:

- **Resectable pancreatic cancer**, defined by imaging as having no distant metastasis or involvement of major vessels.

- **Borderline resectable disease**, where limited vessel involvement may allow for resection after neoadjuvant therapy.
- **Selected cases of locally advanced disease** where tumors respond dramatically to chemotherapy or chemoradiation, allowing for conversion to resectability.

Absolute contraindications to surgery include distant metastases (e.g., liver, lung, peritoneum), extensive vascular encasement not amenable to reconstruction, and poor performance status or comorbidities that prohibit major surgery.

Preoperative Evaluation

A thorough **preoperative workup** is essential to assess tumor resectability, evaluate surgical risk, and prepare the patient for the best possible outcome. This includes:

Imaging Studies

- **Pancreatic protocol CT scan**: Helps delineate the tumor, assess vessel involvement, and detect metastases.
- **MRI/MRCP**: Useful in evaluating the biliary tree and small hepatic metastases.
- **EUS with biopsy**: Confirms diagnosis when tissue sampling is necessary.
- **Staging laparoscopy**: Sometimes used in high-risk patients to rule out

occult metastases before proceeding with laparotomy.

Laboratory Evaluation

- **Complete blood count, renal and liver function tests, coagulation profile**, and **tumor markers** (e.g., CA 19-9).
- **Nutritional assessment** is vital, as many patients are malnourished due to weight loss and anorexia.
- **Cardiopulmonary evaluation** to assess surgical risk.

Biliary Decompression

In patients with **obstructive jaundice**, preoperative biliary drainage may be performed using **endoscopic stenting** if surgery is delayed. However, routine stenting in all patients is not universally recommended due to the risk of infection.

Types of Pancreatic Surgery

1. Pancreaticoduodenectomy (Whipple Procedure)

This is the standard procedure for tumors located in the **head of the pancreas**, periampullary region, or distal bile duct.

Procedure Overview

- Resection includes the **pancreatic head, duodenum, proximal jejunum, gallbladder, common bile duct**, and **distal stomach** (in classic Whipple) or **pylorus-preserving** variant.
- Reconstruction involves anastomosis between the **pancreatic remnant, bile duct**, and **stomach or duodenum** to the jejunum.

Indications

- Resectable tumors of the pancreatic head
- Ampullary cancers

- Distal cholangiocarcinoma

- Duodenal cancers

Challenges

- Technically demanding
- Requires meticulous anastomoses
- Risk of **delayed gastric emptying**, **pancreatic fistula, intra-abdominal abscess**, and **postoperative hemorrhage**

2. Distal Pancreatectomy

Indicated for tumors located in the **body and tail** of the pancreas.

Key Features

- May or may not include **splenectomy**, depending on tumor location and oncologic principles.
- Less technically challenging than a Whipple but associated with higher rates of **postoperative pancreatic fistula** due to transection of the gland.

Laparoscopic/Robotic Distal Pancreatectomy

- Minimally invasive approaches have been increasingly adopted for selected patients.
- Associated with reduced blood loss, shorter hospital stay, and faster recovery.

3. Total Pancreatectomy

Performed when the tumor is **multifocal** or involves both the head and tail of the pancreas.

Implications

- Results in **complete pancreatic insufficiency**:

  - Requires **lifelong insulin** therapy
  - Requires **pancreatic enzyme replacement**

- Rarely performed and reserved for selected cases due to significant metabolic consequences.

4. Vascular Resection and Reconstruction

In **borderline resectable** cases, involvement of the **portal vein or superior mesenteric vein (SMV)** may necessitate **venous resection** with reconstruction using autologous vein grafts or synthetic conduits.

- Arterial resection (SMA or celiac artery) is associated with **higher morbidity and mortality** and is rarely undertaken outside of clinical trials or highly specialized centers.

Intraoperative Considerations

- **Frozen section analysis**: Ensures clear margins during resection.
- **Lymphadenectomy**: Standard procedure includes regional lymph node dissection. Extended lymphadenectomy has not demonstrated a survival benefit.
- **Blood loss control**: Pancreatic surgery can result in significant bleeding; meticulous technique is essential.
- **Operative time**: Whipple procedures may last 5–8 hours depending on complexity.

Postoperative Management

Postoperative care focuses on **monitoring for complications, nutritional support**, and **glycemic control**.

Common Complications

- **Pancreatic fistula**: Leakage from the pancreaticojejunostomy. Managed conservatively in most cases.
- **Delayed gastric emptying**: May require prolonged nasogastric suction and nutritional support.

- **Infection and abscess formation**
  - **Hemorrhage**: Either early (intraoperative) or delayed (pseudoaneurysm rupture).

Nutritional Support

- Patients often require **enteral or parenteral nutrition**.
- Enzyme supplementation may be needed,
  especially after distal or total pancreatectomy.

Glycemic Control

- New-onset or worsening **diabetes mellitus** is common.

- Requires close monitoring and initiation of insulin therapy as needed.

Length of Hospital Stay

- Typically ranges from 7–14 days depending on recovery and complications.
- Enhanced Recovery After Surgery (ERAS) protocols are increasingly adopted to optimize outcomes.

Surgical Outcomes and Survival

Surgical outcomes have improved significantly over the last two decades due to advances in perioperative care and centralization of pancreatic surgery to high-volume centers.

Prognostic Factors

- **Margin status (R0 vs. R1/R2)**: Clear margins (R0) are associated with significantly better survival.
- **Lymph node involvement**: Nodal metastases indicate a poorer prognosis.
- **Tumor grade** and **histological subtype • Response to neoadjuvant therapy**

Survival Statistics

- Median survival for resected pancreatic adenocarcinoma: **18–24 months**

- 5-year survival rates after R0 resection: **15–25%**
- Significantly improved outcomes when surgery is followed by **adjuvant chemotherapy**

Minimally Invasive and Robotic Surgery

Minimally invasive surgery, including **laparoscopic** and **robotic approaches**, has gained traction in pancreatic surgery, particularly for **distal pancreatectomy** and increasingly for selected **Whipple procedures**.

Advantages

- Reduced blood loss
- Shorter recovery time
- Less postoperative pain
- Comparable oncologic outcomes in selected cases

Limitations

- Requires high technical expertise
- Longer operative times
- Limited availability in low-resource settings

Neoadjuvant and Adjuvant Therapies

Neoadjuvant Therapy

Increasingly used in borderline resectable and even resectable cases, neoadjuvant chemotherapy helps by:

- Reducing tumor size
- Assessing biological behavior of the tumor
- Treating micrometastases early

Adjuvant Therapy

Standard practice following surgery for pancreatic adenocarcinoma includes **chemotherapy**, most commonly with **FOLFIRINOX** or **gemcitabine-based regimens**, depending on patient performance status.

Palliative Surgical Procedures

In patients with **unresectable** disease but significant symptoms, surgical palliation may be offered:

- **Biliary bypass** (e.g., hepaticojejunostomy) for obstructive jaundice
- **Gastrojejunostomy** for gastric outlet obstruction
- **Celiac plexus block** for pain management

These interventions can improve quality of life, even if not curative.

generate **Chapter 5: Chemotherapy and Targeted Therapy** in the same structured format.

Chapter 5

Chemotherapy and Targeted Therapy

Chemotherapy and targeted therapy have become central components in the multidisciplinary management of pancreatic cancer. Although pancreatic adenocarcinoma is notoriously resistant to systemic treatment, ongoing advancements in cytotoxic regimens and personalized medicine have provided new avenues for disease control, symptom palliation, and modest improvements in survival.

This chapter provides a comprehensive overview of the role of chemotherapy and targeted agents in both the curative and palliative settings. Topics include chemotherapy strategies in resectable, borderline resectable, locally advanced, and metastatic disease, as well as the emerging importance of biomarker testing and precision oncology.

Overview of Systemic Therapy in Pancreatic Cancer

Pancreatic cancer is often diagnosed at an advanced stage. Consequently, systemic therapy plays a crucial role at nearly every point in the disease trajectory:

- **Adjuvant chemotherapy** is administered after surgical resection to eradicate microscopic disease and reduce recurrence risk.

- **Neoadjuvant therapy** is increasingly used for borderline resectable and locally advanced cases to shrink tumors, increase R0 resection rates, and select for patients who will benefit most from surgery.
- **Primary systemic chemotherapy** is the mainstay of treatment for patients with unresectable or metastatic pancreatic cancer.
- **Targeted therapy** and **immunotherapy** are emerging as important tools in selected patient

subgroups with actionable genetic alterations.

Adjuvant Chemotherapy

Adjuvant chemotherapy is recommended for all patients who have undergone curative-intent resection of pancreatic adenocarcinoma, assuming adequate recovery and performance status. The rationale is based on the high risk of micrometastatic disease and local recurrence even after seemingly complete resection.

Recommended Regimens

1. **Modified FOLFIRINOX**

- A combination of 5-fluorouracil (5-FU), leucovorin, irinotecan, and oxaliplatin.
- Shown to improve disease-free survival and overall survival in the PRODIGE 24/CCTG PA.6 trial.
- Best suited for younger patients with good performance status (ECOG 0–1).

2. **Gemcitabine plus Capecitabine**

- Proven effective in the ESPAC-4 trial, offering a modest survival benefit over gemcitabine monotherapy.
- A reasonable option for patients unable to tolerate FOLFIRINOX.

3. Gemcitabine Monotherapy

○ Still used for patients with borderline performance status or comorbidities precluding combination therapy.

Adjuvant chemotherapy is typically started within 8–12 weeks postoperatively and continued for 6 months, assuming no major toxicity or disease progression.

Neoadjuvant Chemotherapy

Neoadjuvant therapy is used to downstage tumors, increase the likelihood of margin-negative (R0) resection, and identify patients with biologically aggressive disease who may not benefit from surgery.

Indications

- **Borderline resectable tumors** with vascular involvement
- **Locally advanced tumors** that may become resectable after tumor shrinkage
- **Resectable tumors**, in select high-risk patients (e.g., elevated CA 19-9, large tumors)

Common Regimens

- **FOLFIRINOX** is the preferred neoadjuvant regimen due to higher response rates.
- **Gemcitabine with nab-paclitaxel** may be used when FOLFIRINOX is contraindicated.

- Often followed by short-course chemoradiation and restaging imaging.

Outcomes from studies like PREOPANC suggest improved R0 resection rates, lower lymph node involvement, and possibly improved survival with neoadjuvant strategies.

Chemotherapy for Advanced and Metastatic Disease

Most patients with pancreatic cancer are diagnosed at an advanced or metastatic stage, where systemic chemotherapy remains the primary treatment modality.

First-Line Therapy

1. **FOLFIRINOX**

○ Demonstrated superior overall survival (11.1 vs. 6.8 months) compared to gemcitabine in the ACCORD trial.

○ Side effects: neutropenia, diarrhea, fatigue, peripheral neuropathy.

2. **Gemcitabine plus nab-paclitaxel**

○ Shown to prolong survival in the MPACT trial.

○ Side effects: myelosuppression, peripheral neuropathy, alopecia.

3. **Gemcitabine monotherapy**

○ Reserved for elderly or frail patients.

○ Less effective but better tolerated.

Second-Line Therapy

Second-line treatment options are determined by prior therapy and performance status. Common regimens include:

- **Nanoparticle irinotecan (nal-IRI) + 5-FU/leucovorin**
  - **FOLFOX (5-FU + oxaliplatin)** after gemcitabine failure

Targeted Therapy in Pancreatic Cancer

While the majority of pancreatic cancers harbor mutations in genes like **KRAS, TP53**, and **SMAD4**, most of these are currently undruggable. However, a subset of tumors contains **actionable mutations**, which may respond to targeted therapy.

1. PARP Inhibitors

Patients with **germline BRCA1/2 or PALB2** mutations may benefit from **PARP inhibitors** such as **Olaparib**.

- **Mechanism**: Inhibits DNA repair enzymes, leading to synthetic lethality in tumors with defective homologous recombination repair.
- **Indication**: Maintenance therapy after response to platinum-based chemotherapy.

- **Trial evidence**: POLO trial demonstrated prolonged progression-free survival in BRCA-mutated metastatic pancreatic cancer.

2. Immune Checkpoint Inhibitors

Although pancreatic cancer is typically immunologically "cold," a small proportion (<2%) of tumors are **MSI-H** or **dMMR**.

- These tumors may respond to **pembrolizumab**, a PD-1 inhibitor.

- These patients should be identified through **mismatch repair testing** or **MSI profiling**.

3. KRAS Wild-Type Tumors

About 10–15% of pancreatic cancers are **KRAS wild-type**, and these may harbor other actionable alterations such as:

- **NTRK gene fusions**

- **ALK rearrangements • ROS1 mutations**

These tumors may be responsive to corresponding inhibitors like **larotrectinib** (NTRK) or **entrectinib**.

Molecular Profiling and Personalized Medicine

Given the increasing relevance of targeted therapy, **molecular profiling** is now a key step in the diagnostic workup. Testing should include:

- **Next-generation sequencing (NGS)**
- **Germline genetic testing** for BRCA1/2 and other inherited mutations
- **Tumor testing** for MSI status and actionable fusions

This helps identify eligibility for clinical trials and precision-based treatment.

Supportive Care During Chemotherapy

Chemotherapy-related toxicities can impact quality of life and treatment adherence. Proactive management is essential.

Common Adverse Effects

- **Neutropenia and infection**
- **Diarrhea**, particularly with irinotecan
- **Peripheral neuropathy**, from oxaliplatin or paclitaxel
- **Nausea and vomiting**, controlled with antiemetics

- **Fatigue and anorexia**

Nutritional Support

Many patients develop **cachexia** and **exocrine pancreatic insufficiency**, requiring:

- **Pancreatic enzyme replacement therapy (PERT)** • **Nutritional counseling and supplements**
- Appetite stimulants in selected patients

Psychosocial Support

Depression, anxiety, and distress are common in pancreatic cancer patients. Integrating **palliative care** early in the course of treatment improves both symptom control and overall quality of life.

Clinical Trials and Investigational Therapies

Ongoing trials are exploring:

- **Tumor vaccines** (e.g., GVAX, CRS-207)

- **Oncolytic viruses** • **Stromal targeting agents** • **Combination immunotherapy strategies**

All patients, particularly those with advanced disease or rare mutations, should be encouraged to consider participation in **clinical trials** to access novel agents and contribute to research.

Chapter 6

Radiation Therapy in Pancreatic Cancer

Introduction
Radiation therapy has emerged as a key component in the multidisciplinary

management of pancreatic cancer. Although pancreatic tumors have historically been considered resistant to radiation, recent technological advances and improved understanding of tumor biology have broadened the applications of radiotherapy. As a locoregional treatment, radiation therapy plays a significant role in enhancing local control, increasing surgical resectability, reducing recurrence, and alleviating symptoms in palliative cases. This chapter explores the indications, techniques, and outcomes of radiation therapy in pancreatic cancer, highlighting evidence-based practices and emerging innovations.

Radiation Therapy Modalities in Pancreatic Cancer Several types of radiation therapy are utilized in treating pancreatic cancer, each with unique mechanisms and applications:

- **External Beam Radiation Therapy (EBRT)**: This traditional method involves delivering radiation from an external source directed at the tumor site. EBRT has been the backbone of radiation therapy in oncology and remains widely used in pancreatic cancer.

- **Three-Dimensional Conformal Radiation Therapy (3D-CRT)**: An improvement over conventional EBRT, 3D-CRT uses imaging to shape the radiation beams to the tumor's geometry, reducing exposure to surrounding healthy tissue.

- **Intensity-Modulated Radiation Therapy**
    (IMRT): A more advanced version of EBRT, IMRT allows for varying intensities within individual beams, enabling highly conformal dose distributions. This technique minimizes radiation dose to adjacent organs like the duodenum, stomach, kidneys, and spinal cord.

- **Stereotactic Body Radiation Therapy (SBRT)**: SBRT delivers high doses of focused radiation over a few fractions. Its precision makes it ideal for treating small, localized pancreatic tumors. SBRT is typically used in the neoadjuvant or definitive setting when surgery is not an immediate option.

- **Proton Beam Therapy**: Proton therapy offers dosimetric advantages due to the Bragg peak phenomenon, where the radiation dose is deposited within the tumor with minimal exit dose. While promising, its use in pancreatic cancer remains limited and under investigation.

Clinical Indications

Radiation therapy is applied in several clinical contexts for pancreatic cancer:

1. **Neoadjuvant Therapy**: In borderline resectable or locally advanced cases, preoperative radiation (often combined with chemotherapy) can shrink the tumor, facilitate surgical

resection, and increase R0 resection rates.

2. **Definitive Therapy**: For patients with locally advanced, unresectable pancreatic cancer (LAPC), radiation therapy is used to control local disease progression, especially when the disease is confined but not operable.

3. **Adjuvant Therapy**: Postoperative radiation may be considered for patients with positive surgical margins (R1) or extensive nodal involvement, aiming to eradicate residual microscopic disease.

4. **Palliative Therapy**: In patients with advanced or metastatic disease experiencing pain, biliary obstruction, or gastrointestinal bleeding, short-

course radiation can relieve symptoms and improve quality of life.

Treatment Planning and Simulation
Successful radiation therapy relies on meticulous planning:

- **Simulation**: Patients undergo CT simulation in treatment position. Immobilization devices and contrast-enhanced imaging may be used. PET and MRI may be fused with CT for better tumor delineation.

- **Target Volume Definition**:

    o Gross Tumor Volume (GTV): Identified tumor based on imaging.
    o Clinical Target Volume (CTV): GTV plus margin to account for microscopic disease.

○ Planning Target Volume (PTV): CTV plus margin for daily setup and organ motion variability.

- **Organ-at-Risk (OAR) Contouring**: Nearby structures such as the liver, kidneys, bowel, spinal cord, and stomach are contoured to limit radiation exposure.

- **Motion Management**: Respiratory-induced tumor motion is a significant challenge in abdominal radiotherapy. Techniques include:

  0 Respiratory gating
  ○ Abdominal compression
  ○ Breath-hold techniques (e.g., deep inspiration breath-hold)
  ○ Four-dimensional CT (4D-CT)

Radiation Dose and Fractionation

Doses vary depending on the intent of therapy:

- **Neoadjuvant/Adjuvant EBRT**: Typically delivered in 25–28 fractions, totaling 45–54 Gy over 5–6 weeks.
- **Definitive Chemoradiation**: Similar dose range with concurrent chemotherapy.
- **SBRT**: High-dose radiation (25–40 Gy) over 3–5 fractions.
- **Palliative Radiation**: Short-course schedules, such as 30 Gy in 10 fractions or 20 Gy in 5 fractions.

Concurrent Chemoradiation

Combining radiation with chemotherapy enhances the cytotoxic effects of both modalities. Common radiosensitizing agents include:

- 5-Fluorouracil (5-FU)

- Capecitabine
- Gemcitabine

Chemoradiation is particularly effective in downstaging tumors and improving local control in unresectable cases. Careful patient monitoring is required due to increased toxicity.

Clinical Evidence and Trials
The role of radiation therapy in pancreatic cancer has evolved through multiple studies:

- **Gastrointestinal Tumor Study Group (GITSG) Trial (1985)**: Demonstrated a survival advantage for patients receiving postoperative chemoradiation.

- **EORTC 40891 Trial**: Questioned the benefit of adjuvant chemoradiation, showing no significant improvement in overall survival.

- **RTOG 9704**: Evaluated gemcitabine-based chemoradiation and showed improved local control, though survival benefits were marginal.

- **PREOPANC Trial (Dutch Study)**: Provided evidence for neoadjuvant chemoradiation improving disease-free survival and R0 resection rates compared to immediate surgery.

- **LAP07 Trial**: Focused on LAPC and found chemoradiation delayed local progression but did not significantly improve survival.

Emerging studies continue to investigate the value of dose escalation, integration with immunotherapy, and new fractionation schedules.

Side Effects and Toxicity Management
Radiation side effects can be categorized as acute or late:

- **Acute Effects**:

    - Nausea, vomiting
    - Fatigue
    - Anorexia
    - Diarrhea
    - Epigastric discomfort

- **Late Effects**:

- Gastrointestinal ulcers or bleeding
- Biliary strictures
- Renal impairment
- Hepatotoxicity
- Second malignancies (rare)

Supportive measures include nutritional support, antiemetics, hydration, and close monitoring of organ function. Modern techniques like IMRT and SBRT have substantially reduced the risk of severe toxicity.

Patient Selection Criteria

Selecting appropriate candidates is essential to maximize benefit and minimize harm:

- **Performance Status**: ECOG 0–2 preferred
- **Tumor Location and Vascular Involvement**

• Absence of Widespread Metastasis • Patient Preferences and Comorbidities

Patients must be assessed through multidisciplinary team discussions, incorporating input from surgical oncology, medical oncology, radiation oncology, radiology, and pathology.

Special Considerations

- **Elderly Patients**: Treatment must be individualized based on functional status, not age alone.
- **Prior Abdominal Radiation**: Reirradiation may be possible with advanced techniques like MRgRT and proton therapy.
- **Genomic Variants**: Patients with BRCA mutations or other DNA repair gene deficiencies may respond differently to radiation.

Advancements and Emerging Technologies

- **MRI-Guided Radiation Therapy (MRgRT)**: Enables real-time tumor tracking and adaptive planning. Improves soft tissue visualization and treatment precision.

- **Proton Therapy**: Under trial for its tissue-sparing properties. May benefit patients with tumors near radiosensitive organs.
- **Radiogenomics**: Investigates correlations between genetic profiles and radiation response.

- **Artificial Intelligence (AI)**: AI-assisted planning can enhance target delineation, automate planning, and predict toxicity.

- **Biologically Guided Radiation Therapy (BGRT)**: Uses functional imaging like PET to guide dose painting and personalize treatment.

Future Directions

Several promising avenues are being explored:

- **Immuno-Radiotherapy**: Radiation can increase tumor immunogenicity. Trials are assessing its combination with immune checkpoint inhibitors.
- **Dose Escalation Trials**: Aiming to increase local control without compromising safety.

- **Personalized Radiation**: Leveraging genomic and imaging biomarkers to guide dose and technique.
- **Short-Course vs. Long-Course Radiation**: Ongoing debate and trials to determine optimal schedules.

Chapter 7

Palliative Care in Pancreatic Cancer

Introduction
Pancreatic cancer is a highly aggressive malignancy with a poor prognosis. Given its

late presentation and limited curative treatment options, a large proportion of patients are not eligible for surgery or long-term disease control. In this context, palliative care becomes a central component of comprehensive cancer management. Palliative care in pancreatic cancer focuses not only on physical symptom control but also on psychological, social, and spiritual aspects, aiming to improve quality of life for both patients and their families. This chapter explores the principles, interventions, and multidisciplinary approach of palliative care in pancreatic cancer.

Principles of Palliative Care

Palliative care is guided by a set of principles that distinguish it from curative treatment:

- **Holistic Approach**: It addresses physical, emotional, social, and spiritual suffering.
- **Patient-Centered**: Care is tailored to the individual goals, preferences, and values of each patient.
- **Early Integration**: Initiating palliative care alongside active treatment improves symptom management and quality of life.
- **Team-Based**: Involves physicians, nurses, psychologists, social workers, chaplains, and allied professionals.
- **Continuity of Care**: Encompasses all stages of the disease, including end-of-life care and bereavement support for families.

Common Symptoms in Pancreatic Cancer

Patients with pancreatic cancer commonly suffer from multiple, often severe symptoms. Timely and effective management of these symptoms is crucial.

1. **Pain**
    - Caused by tumor invasion of nerves, organs, and surrounding tissues.
    - Often manifests as epigastric or back pain.
    - Management includes:
        - WHO pain ladder (non-opioids → weak opioids → strong opioids).
        - Nerve blocks (e.g., celiac plexus block).
        - Adjuncts like antidepressants or anticonvulsants for neuropathic pain.
2. **Obstructive Jaundice**

    - Due to tumor compression of the common bile duct.

- Presents with pruritus, dark urine, pale stools, and liver dysfunction.
- Management:
    - Endoscopic biliary stenting (plastic or metal).
    - Percutaneous transhepatic biliary drainage
    - Surgical bypass in selected cases.

3. **Gastrointestinal Obstruction**
   - Can involve the duodenum or stomach.
   - Symptoms include nausea, vomiting, and early satiety.
   - Treatment:
       - Endoscopic stent placement.
       - Gastrojejunostomy surgery for longer survival.

- Antiemetics and nutritional support.

4. Cachexia and Weight Loss

- Multifactorial: decreased intake, malabsorption, systemic inflammation.
- Management:

  - Nutritional counseling and calorie supplementation.
  - Pancreatic enzyme replacement therapy (PERT).
  - Appetite stimulants like megestrol acetate or corticosteroids.

5. Fatigue and Weakness

- Profound and often distressing.
- Address reversible causes: anemia, infection, depression.

- Encourage activity within limits; energy conservation techniques.

6. Psychological Distress

- Depression and anxiety are common.
  - Psychosocial support, counseling, pharmacotherapy.
  - Support groups and spiritual care as needed.

7. Ascites and Fluid Retention

- Occurs in advanced disease stages.
- Managed with diuretics, paracentesis, and salt restriction.

Communication and Prognostic Discussions

Effective communication is a cornerstone of palliative care. Conversations about prognosis, goals of care, and treatment options must be handled with empathy and clarity.

- Use the "Ask-Tell-Ask" framework.
- Provide information in small, digestible segments.
- Explore patient understanding and expectations.
- Offer hope while remaining honest.
- Involve family in decision-making.
- Document and revisit care preferences regularly.

Advance Care Planning (ACP)
ACP enables patients to make informed decisions about their future care, especially in the event of cognitive decline or clinical deterioration.
- Components:
    - Advance directives (e.g., living wills).
    - Durable power of attorney for healthcare.

- o Do-not-resuscitate (DNR) orders.
- Benefits:
  - o Reduces unwanted interventions.
    - o Improves end-of-life care consistency with patient wishes.
  - o Lessens caregiver burden and stress.

End-of-Life Care

The terminal phase of pancreatic cancer requires special attention to comfort and dignity.

- **Hospice Care**: Provides palliative care for patients with a life expectancy of less than six months. Services include pain control, nursing care, and emotional support.

- **Home-Based Care**: Often preferred by patients; requires coordination of

medications, equipment, and
caregiver support.
- **Symptom Management**:
  - ○ Use of opioids for pain and
  dyspnea.
  - ○ Anxiolytics for restlessness.
  - ○ Anticholinergics for secretion
  control.
  - ○ Avoid aggressive, non-beneficial
  treatments.

Multidisciplinary Palliative Care Team
Successful palliative care depends on
collaboration among various professionals:

- **Palliative Care Physician**: Leads
  symptom management and
  coordinates care.
- **Oncologist**: Guides disease-specific
  treatment decisions.
- **Nurse/Nurse Practitioner**: Provides
  bedside care and education.

- **Social Worker**: Assists with resources, family counseling, financial and housing issues.
- **Psychologist or Psychiatrist**: Supports mental health and coping.
- **Chaplains/Spiritual Counselors**: Address spiritual suffering and existential distress.
- **Nutritionist**: Helps manage diet, cachexia, and GI symptoms.

Integrating Palliative Care with Oncology Early integration of palliative care alongside standard oncologic care leads to improved patient outcomes.

- Studies show improved quality of life, better symptom control, and reduced depression.
- Patients receiving early palliative care may live longer.

- Encourages appropriate use of hospice and fewer aggressive interventions at end of life.

Cultural and Ethical Considerations
Palliative care must be respectful of diverse cultural beliefs and ethical values.

- **Cultural Sensitivity**:

  o Respect for different attitudes toward disclosure, decision-making, and death.
  o Inclusion of family and community figures when appropriate.
- **Ethical Principles**:

o Autonomy: Honoring patient
preferences.

o Beneficence and non-
maleficence:
Providing benefit and avoiding
harm.
o Justice: Equitable access to
palliative care.

Financial and Logistical Barriers

Barriers to palliative care access and
delivery in pancreatic cancer include:

- High treatment costs and limited
  insurance coverage.
- Shortage of trained palliative care
  providers.
- Inadequate infrastructure for home-
  based or rural palliative services.
- Patient and caregiver misconceptions
  about palliative care.

Solutions include:

- Health policy reforms.
- Expansion of community-based palliative services.
- Public education campaigns.
- Telemedicine and mobile health units for remote areas.

Role of Caregivers

Caregivers play an essential role in the care of patients with advanced pancreatic cancer. They provide physical, emotional, and logistical support.

- Common caregiver challenges:
  - Emotional stress and burnout.
  - Financial strain.

- ○ Navigating complex care decisions.
- • Support strategies:
  - o Caregiver training and education.
  - ○ Respite care services.
  - ○ Psychological support and counseling.
- ○ Inclusion in care planning and decision-making.

Grief and Bereavement Support

Bereavement care is often overlooked but vital in the continuum of palliative care.

- • Services include:
  - ○ Grief counseling.
  - ○ Support groups.
  - ○ Memorial services

- • High-risk groups (e.g., spouses, children, isolated individuals) may require more intensive support.

- Institutions should offer structured bereavement programs for at least 13 months post-loss.

Innovations in Palliative Care
New models and tools are improving palliative care delivery in pancreatic cancer:

- **Telepalliative Care**: Remote consultations via video calls, improving access.
- **Prognostic Tools**: Use of predictive algorithms to identify patients needing early palliative intervention.
- **Mobile Apps**: For symptom tracking, medication reminders, and patient education.
- **Integration of AI**: To personalize palliative interventions and predict symptom trajectories

Chapter 8
Future Directions in the Management of Pancreatic Cancer

Introduction

Pancreatic cancer remains one of the most formidable malignancies in oncology, characterized by late diagnosis, aggressive progression, limited response to traditional therapies, and a low five-year survival rate. While significant progress has been made in understanding its pathogenesis and treatment, the future of pancreatic cancer management lies in a multidisciplinary and innovative approach encompassing advances in molecular biology, early detection, targeted therapies, immunotherapy, artificial intelligence, personalized medicine, and public health initiatives. This chapter provides a comprehensive overview of the most promising future directions in the fight against pancreatic cancer.

Advancements in Early Detection and Diagnosis Early detection of pancreatic cancer significantly increases the chance of curative treatment. Future strategies are focused on improving diagnostic tools for identifying the disease in its earliest stages.

1. **Biomarkers**

   - Current biomarkers like CA 19-9 lack sufficient sensitivity and specificity.

- Ongoing research focuses on discovering novel biomarkers:
  - Circulating tumor DNA (ctDNA).
    - Exosomes containing pancreatic cancer-specific RNA and proteins.
- MicroRNAs (miRNAs) detectable in blood, saliva, or urine.
- DNA methylation patterns linked to malignancy.
  - Multiplex assays and biomarker panels are being developed to improve diagnostic accuracy.

2. **Imaging Innovations**

- Artificial intelligence (AI) algorithms are enhancing the detection of pancreatic lesions on CT, MRI, and endoscopic ultrasound.

- Molecular imaging techniques such as PET-MRI using specific tracers are under investigation.
- Contrast-enhanced harmonic endoscopic ultrasound (CEH-EUS) allows better visualization of vascular patterns.

3. Screening High-Risk Populations

- Genetic screening for BRCA mutations, CDKN2A, and STK11/LKB1 is identifying individuals at higher risk.
- Surveillance programs with periodic EUS and MRI in genetically predisposed individuals are becoming more common.
- Development of low-cost, non-invasive blood tests for broad population screening is a critical research area.

Molecular and Genetic Insights

A deeper understanding of pancreatic cancer biology is essential for developing effective treatments.

1. Molecular Subtyping

- Pancreatic cancers are now classified into molecular subtypes such as basal-like and classical.
- Molecular profiling helps predict response to chemotherapy and targeted agents.
- Future protocols may incorporate subtype-based therapeutic strategies.

2. Genomic Alterations

- Common mutations include KRAS, TP53, CDKN2A, and SMAD4.
- Next-generation sequencing (NGS) panels are used to identify actionable mutations.
- Precision oncology initiatives focus on matching patients with therapies targeting specific mutations.

3. Organoid Models and Tumor-on-a-Chip

- Patient-derived organoids allow ex vivo testing of drug responses.
- Tumor-on-a-chip models recreate the tumor microenvironment, enabling

drug screening and mechanistic studies.

Innovative Systemic Therapies
Despite advances in surgery and radiation, systemic therapies remain the cornerstone of treatment for most pancreatic cancer patients.

1. **Targeted Therapy**

   o **PARP Inhibitors**: Beneficial in patients with BRCA mutations (e.g., olaparib).
   o **NTRK Inhibitors**: For patients with NTRK gene fusions.
   o **KRAS Inhibitors**: Emerging agents like sotorasib targeting specific KRAS mutations.
   o Efforts continue to target the tumor stroma and desmoplastic reaction.

2. Immunotherapy

- Pancreatic cancer is typically resistant to immune checkpoint inhibitors.
- Future strategies include:

    - Combination therapies (e.g., checkpoint inhibitors with chemotherapy or radiation).
    - Cancer vaccines (e.g., GVAX, KRAS-targeted vaccines).
    - Adoptive T-cell therapy (e.g., CAR-T cells specific to pancreatic tumor antigens).

- Oncolytic viruses
  engineered to
  selectively infect and
  destroy tumor cells.

3. **Nanomedicine**

  ○ Nanoformulations improve
  drug delivery and reduce
  toxicity.
  ○ Liposomal irinotecan and
  nanoparticle albumin-bound
  paclitaxel are examples.
  ○ Future designs include smart
  nanoparticles that respond to
  the tumor microenvironment.

Advances in Surgical Techniques
Surgery offers the only potential cure for
pancreatic cancer, but future developments
aim to improve outcomes and expand
eligibility.

1. Minimally Invasive and Robotic Surgery

- ○ Robotic pancreatoduodenectomy offers greater precision and shorter recovery.
- ○ Laparoscopic surgery is gaining traction for selected tumors.

2. Intraoperative Imaging

- ○ Fluorescence-guided surgery using tumor-specific dyes enhances margin clearance.
- ○ Real-time molecular imaging may help detect micrometastases.

3. Neoadjuvant and Adjuvant Innovations

- More effective neoadjuvant protocols using FOLFIRINOX and chemoradiotherapy.
- Integration of molecular profiling into preoperative decision-making.

Radiotherapy Evolution

Radiation therapy is evolving into a more precise and effective modality.

1. Stereotactic Body Radiation Therapy (SBRT)

- High-dose, focused radiation in fewer sessions.
- Well-tolerated with promising local control.

2. Proton Beam Therapy

○ Reduces damage to surrounding tissues.

○ May be suitable for tumors near critical structures.

3. Biologically Guided Radiotherapy

○ Uses tumor metabolic activity (e.g., from PET scans) to guide dosing.

○ Adaptive radiotherapy systems adjust treatment in real time.

Artificial Intelligence and Big Data
AI and big data are transforming cancer care through prediction, personalization, and decision support.

1. Predictive Analytics
○ Machine learning models predict survival, recurrence, and treatment response.

- Natural language processing (NLP) analyzes electronic health records for insights.

2. Radiomics and Pathomics

- Extracts large-scale data from imaging and pathology slides.
- Assists in diagnosis, prognosis, and therapy selection.

3. Clinical Decision Support Tools

- AI-powered platforms guide clinicians on therapy choices based on real-time data.

4. Data Sharing and Registries

- Global initiatives like The Cancer Genome Atlas (TCGA) and AACR GENIE are pooling data to accelerate discovery.

Personalized and Precision Medicine
The era of precision medicine aims to tailor treatments to the individual patient's tumor biology.

1. **Molecular Tumor Boards**
   ○ Interdisciplinary teams review genomic data to personalize treatment plans.
2. **Liquid Biopsies**

   ○ Non-invasive monitoring of tumor DNA and RNA in the blood.
   ○ Detect recurrence and treatment resistance early.
3. **Theranostics**
   ○ Combines diagnostic and therapeutic capabilities in a single agent.
   ○ Examples include radiolabeled peptides for imaging and therapy.

Psychosocial and Supportive Innovations

Improving quality of life is as important as extending it.

1. **Digital Health Tools**
   - Mobile apps for symptom tracking, medication adherence, and communication.
   - Virtual reality (VR) for distraction during procedures or relaxation.
2. **Telehealth Expansion**

   - Improves access to oncology and palliative care, especially in rural areas.
3. **Patient Navigation and Advocacy**

   - Professional navigators help patients manage appointments, treatments, and insurance.
   - Empowerment through patient education and community support.

Global Health and Policy Implications

Global collaboration and policy reform are essential for equitable progress.

1. **Access to Care**

   - Efforts to reduce disparities in diagnosis and treatment.
   - Expansion of universal healthcare and insurance coverage.

2. **Research Funding and Policy**

   - Increased investment in pancreatic cancer research.
   - Incentives for orphan drug development.

3. **Awareness and Education**

   - Public campaigns to raise awareness of symptoms and risk factors.

○ Education of healthcare providers on updated screening guidelines.

Future Clinical Trials and Collaborative Models Clinical research is vital for future advancements.

1. **Basket and Umbrella Trials**

   ○ Match patients to therapies based on genetic alterations rather than tumor type.

2. **Platform Trials**

   ○ Allow multiple therapies to be tested simultaneously with shared controls.

3. Patient-Centered Outcomes

○ Increasing emphasis on quality of life, functional status, and patient preferences.

4. Global Consortia

○ Initiatives like Precision Promise (Lustgarten Foundation) aim to accelerate innovation.

Chapter 9

Integrative and Supportive Therapies in Pancreatic Cancer Management

Introduction

Pancreatic cancer is a highly aggressive malignancy with a dismal prognosis and significant treatment-related morbidity. The physical and psychological toll of the disease often extends beyond the capabilities of conventional therapies, necessitating an integrative approach. Integrative and supportive therapies encompass a broad range of modalities that aim to improve quality of life, reduce symptoms, support mental health, and complement standard treatments such as surgery, chemotherapy, and radiation. These therapies range from evidence-based complementary medicine and nutritional interventions to psychosocial support, physical rehabilitation, and spiritual care. In this chapter, we explore the critical role of integrative and supportive therapies in the holistic management of pancreatic cancer.

Defining Integrative Oncology
Integrative oncology is an evidence-informed, patient-centered field that combines conventional cancer treatments with complementary therapies to address physical, emotional, and spiritual needs.

1. **Principles of Integrative Oncology**

   o Whole-person care: addressing body, mind, and spirit.

○ Informed decision-making between patients and providers.
○ Evidence-based application of complementary therapies.
○ Promotion of health, wellness, and survivorship.

2. Scope in Pancreatic Cancer

○ Symptom control: pain, nausea, fatigue.
○ Psychological support: anxiety, depression.

- Nutritional counseling and physical rehabilitation.
- Spiritual well-being and quality of life.

Nutritional Support and Counseling

Malnutrition is a prevalent concern in pancreatic cancer patients due to anorexia, treatment side effects, and exocrine pancreatic insufficiency.

1. **Nutritional Challenges**

o Weight loss, muscle wasting (cachexia). o Malabsorption and steatorrhea.

   o Diabetes mellitus from pancreatic endocrine insufficiency.

2. Nutritional Interventions

   o Dietitian-led counseling tailored to treatment phases. High-protein, high-calorie diets.

   o Pancreatic enzyme replacement therapy (PERT).

   o

- Nutritional supplements (e.g., omega-3 fatty acids, vitamin D).
- Enteral nutrition in advanced cases.

3. **Role of Nutraceuticals**

- Curcumin, green tea polyphenols, resveratrol: investigated for anti-inflammatory and anti-cancer properties.
- Caution advised due to limited clinical evidence and potential drug interactions.

Pain and Symptom Management

Pain, fatigue, and gastrointestinal symptoms are commonly reported and significantly impair quality of life.

1. **Pain Management**

   - WHO analgesic ladder: non-opioids, weak opioids, strong opioids.
   - Celiac plexus block for refractory abdominal pain.
   - Neuropathic pain agents: gabapentin, pregabalin.
   - Integrative options: acupuncture, massage therapy.

2. **Management of Gastrointestinal Symptoms**

   -

    ○ Antiemetics for nausea
      (ondansetron, dexamethasone).
    ○ Antidiarrheals and stool
    softeners. ○ Antispasmodics
    for cramping.
    ○ Probiotics for gut flora
    modulation.

3. **Fatigue**

    ○ Regular physical activity as
    tolerated.
    ○ Energy conservation techniques.
      Cognitive-behavioral therapy
      (CBT).

Psychological and Emotional Support
Psychological distress is common and often under-addressed in pancreatic cancer care.

1. Prevalence of Psychological Distress

- Up to 40% of patients report anxiety and depression.
- Emotional burden impacts adherence, quality of life, and survival.

2. Psychological Interventions

- Individual or group counseling.
- Support groups tailored to cancer type.

-

○ CBT and mindfulness-based stress reduction (MBSR).

○ Psychiatric medications when indicated.

3. **Role of Psychosocial Oncology**

○ Multidisciplinary collaboration between psychologists, social workers, and oncologists.

○ Screening tools like the Distress Thermometer for early identification.

Mind-Body Medicine

Mind-body practices foster psychological resilience and modulate physiological stress responses.

1. **Meditation and Mindfulness**

○ Proven benefits in reducing anxiety, depression, and pain.

- Techniques: guided imagery, deep breathing, progressive muscle relaxation.

2. **Yoga and Tai Chi**

   - Improve flexibility, strength, and mood. Adaptable for varying levels of physical capacity.

3. **Biofeedback and Hypnotherapy**

   - Promote relaxation and control over physiological symptoms.

   -

○ Useful for pain, nausea, and sleep disturbances.

Complementary Therapies with Scientific Support Some complementary therapies have demonstrated efficacy in controlled studies.

1. **Acupuncture**

   ○ Effective for pain, chemotherapy-induced nausea, and neuropathy.
   ○ Must be administered by trained practitioners in sterile conditions.

2. **Massage Therapy**

   ○ Reduces pain, anxiety, and fatigue.

○ Avoided in thrombocytopenic or cachectic patients.

3. Aromatherapy and Essential Oils

○ May help with relaxation and sleep.
○ Lavender and peppermint are commonly used.

Spiritual and Existential Care
A cancer diagnosis often triggers existential questions and spiritual distress.

1. Assessment of Spiritual Needs

- Tools: FICA (Faith, Importance, Community, Address in care).
- Integration into routine care planning.

2. Spiritual Interventions

- Chaplaincy services.
- Life review and dignity therapy.

- Meditation and religious rituals.

3. Benefits

- Improved coping, peace of mind, and sense of purpose.

- Associated with better patient satisfaction and end-of-life decision-making.

Rehabilitation and Physical Activity
Maintaining physical function enhances independence and psychological health.

1. Exercise Oncology

- Supervised exercise reduces fatigue and improves function.
- Resistance training preserves muscle mass.

2. Rehabilitation Programs

○ Address deconditioning,
balance issues, and mobility.
○ Include physiotherapists,
occupational therapists, and
kinesiologists.

3. **Lymphedema Management**

○ Compression garments,
massage, and exercise for
patients with surgical
complications.

Integrative Care Delivery Models
Successful integration of supportive
therapies requires systemic implementation.

1. **Dedicated Integrative Oncology
Clinics**

○ Multidisciplinary teams: oncologists, naturopaths, psychologists, dietitians.
○ Offer coordinated, evidence-based complementary care.

2. Standardized Assessment Tools

○ PROMIS (Patient-Reported Outcomes Measurement Information System).
○ Edmonton Symptom Assessment System (ESAS).

3. Education and Training

○ Oncology providers need training in integrative approaches.
○ Certification programs in integrative medicine and oncology.

Patient and Caregiver Empowerment
Empowering patients and caregivers improves adherence, satisfaction, and outcomes.

1. **Shared Decision-Making**

○ Informed choices about supportive therapies.

○ Incorporation of patient values and preferences.

2. **Caregiver Support**

○ Educational materials, support groups, and respite care.
○ Psychological counseling for caregiver burden.

3. **Patient Portals and Digital Tools**

○ Track symptoms and communicate with care teams.
○ Access to educational resources and support communities.

Challenges and Ethical Considerations

Despite its benefits, integrative oncology poses certain challenges.

1. Scientific Rigor and Evidence Base

- Need for more randomized controlled trials.
    - Risk of pseudoscience and misinformation.

2. Regulation and Quality Control

- Oversight of supplements and alternative practitioners.
- Accreditation and licensure requirements.

3. Cost and Accessibility

- Insurance coverage for integrative services is limited.
- Programs must be equitable and inclusive.

Conclusion

Pancreatic cancer remains one of the most challenging malignancies in modern medicine, marked by late diagnosis, aggressive progression, and limited treatment options. However, with advances in early detection, precision therapies, and multidisciplinary care, the outlook is gradually improving.

Throughout this book, we have explored the full spectrum of pancreatic cancer management—from diagnostic tools and surgical approaches to chemotherapy, palliative care, and integrative therapies. Each component plays a critical role in improving patient outcomes and quality of life. The integration of supportive care, patient-centered approaches, and emerging technologies represents the future of personalized oncology.

Moving forward, a strong emphasis on early detection, genetic profiling, and innovative therapies will be essential. By continuing to embrace holistic, evidence-based strategies and fostering collaboration across specialties, we can offer pancreatic cancer patients not just longer survival but better lives